Brain Supplements: Everything You N
to Improve Memory, Cognition

GW01457995

TABLE OF CONTENTS

Disclaimer

Please note that I'm not a physician or nutritionist. I've consulted with several, done tons of research and experimentation, but do not claim to be a medical professional. Your health is incredibly precious and you should make informed decisions based on thorough research. Before starting any new diet and exercise program please check with your doctor and clear any exercise and/or diet changes with them before beginning. I am not a doctor or registered dietitian. I do not claim to cure any cause, condition or disease. I do not provide medical aid or nutrition for the purpose of health or disease and claim to be a doctor or dietitian.

I wrote this book because I couldn't find any reliable sources of information out there about nootropics. The information held in this book is merely the opinion and collected research of a layman individual. The research and information covered is open to public domain for discussion and in no way breaches or breaks the boundaries of the law in any state of the United States of America where I live. I am not a doctor nor do I claim to have any formal medical background. I am not liable, either expressly or in an implied manner, nor claim any responsibility for any emotional or physical problems that may occur directly or indirectly from reading this book.

To get a free audio version of this book, visit http://thenootropicsbook.com/audio. I'll also send you a list of approved nootropics suppliers, as well as the latest nootropics research.

Introduction

If you've seen the film *Limitless*, you've probably been attracted to the idea of a pill that allows you to perform tasks far beyond your normal ability. In today's world of constant connection to social media, email and other sources of continual stimulation rewires our brains, many would love to get their hands on a pill that would help them process all they encounter in a given day. Heck, many people would love just to remember all their passwords on different sites.

Millions love to find a pill, supplement or magic food that

helps them to think more clearly, multi-task without breaking a sweat and accelerate their climb up the career ladder. Some need help simply hanging on to their current position, especially as they age and see young people accustomed to multi-tasking coming up through the ranks.

Others, particularly students, are buying smart drugs that enable them to cram for hours on end while retaining every scribble in their notebooks. It's no secret that students have experimented for years with substances that provide an energy boost and aid in concentration and retention, enabling the brain to work longer and harder. These substances are perfect for cramming before an exam, or providing a needed stimulant to crank out a last-minute term paper.

Does such a wonder drug exist, one that can take our brains to a higher level? Could our cognitive function someday rival Bradley Cooper's in *Limitless*? Are there substances out there that can improve our memory, cognition and mental performance? If so, what are they? Are they safe to use?

In this book, we'll cover these brain supplements – collectively known as Nootropics – and show you their history, how they work, and help you understand how to boost your memory and mental performance. Nootropics are a rapidly developing area of nutrition research, and new studies and substances are coming out all the time. To keep up to date with the latest happenings in nootropics world, sign up for my free monthly research newsletter at http://thenootropicsbook.com. Let's dive in!

What Are Nootropics?

The quest to enhance our brainpower has existed for centuries. Thousands of years ago, the Chinese used ginseng, ginkgo biloba and gotu kola extracts to improve their brain function. The discovery of tea's stimulating powers also began about two millennia ago, again in China. Science has indeed verified some of the positive properties of tea and caffeine's role in alertness, but recent years have brought a whole new level of brain studies. Researchers have learned an amazing amount about the brain, and companies and individuals are applying this science to increase our cognitive capabilities.

The web is full of claims for various substances that reportedly help with brain function. This book will help you to sort through those claims and understand the new class of drugs – nootropics – that enhance cognition by increasing memory, boosting concentration, increasing motivation, improving the user's mood and enhancing one's ability to focus.

This new class of drugs is known as "nootropics" (pronounced "new-tropics"), "smart drugs" or "cognitive enhancers." Nootropics work by altering the brain's balance of chemicals in a way that leads to improved mental performance. Many users of these drugs report they are able to focus better, remember more information and keep their brains running at high levels for extended periods of time.

What makes nootropics different from other cognitive enhancers (like caffeine and nicotine) is that they have few side effects and are non-addictive. The criterion that anything termed a nootropic should not have significant side effects removes many stimulants and sedatives (LSD, many amphetamines) from this drug category. Adderall, for instance, is often prescribed for ADHD and gulped down in large quantities by students at exam time, but its side effects keep it from being categorized as a nootropic.

Nootropics research has been ongoing for decades, with most of the breakthroughs coming in the 1970s. Dr. Corneliu Giurgea, a Romanian scientist who synthesized Piracetam (one of the original nootropics which we'll cover shortly) in 1964, first coined the term "Nootropics" in by combining the Greek words for "mind," *noos*, and "to turn or to bend," *trepein*. Thus, the idea is that nootropics bend the mind in a positive way. Dr. Giurgea defined the nootropics category by establishing strict criteria to distinguish these drugs from other stimulants, sedatives and mood-enhancers. Among the criteria that he laid out were that:

- A substance must enhance memory and the ability to learn.

- It must help the brain function under disruptive conditions, such as low oxygen or shock.

- It must protect the brain from chemical and physical assaults, as from certain drugs.

- It must increase the ability of neuronal firing control mechanisms.

- It must lack a significant sedative or stimulatory effect.

- It must have few or no other side effects.

- It must be non-toxic.

These strict criteria ruled out substances like caffeine (due to its significant stimulatory effects) and restricted the type of drugs he would lump under the nootropics category. Nootropics are also different than most cognitive enhancers in that they will produce a measurable improvement in brain function over an extended time period: true nootropics won't become less effective the more you use them. Caffeine does indeed enhance cognitive function, for instance, but only over short periods of time. It also acts as a stimulant, and becomes less effective when used repeatedly over a prolonged period of time, a weakness that keeps it out of the nootropic category.

Many natural and synthetic substances increase cognitive function (and can even repair the brain), but most have side effects or lose their effectiveness over time. In short, all nootropics fall into the category of brain supplements, but not all brain supplements should be labeled nootropics. Nootropics are simply a subset of a larger group of cognitive-enhancing substances.

This book will examine both classical nootropics and other brain supplements, even if some newer products have not been thoroughly vetted for side effects and/or addictive properties. Dozens and dozens of substances are called nootropics on the Internet, but only a few are considered true nootropics, with an even smaller subset fulfilling Dr. Giurgea's criteria.

The most common nootropic drugs are Racetams and their derivatives (with names like Piracetam, Aniracetam, Oxiracetam, Pramiracetam, Noopept), Nuvigil, Provigil, and Choline supplements (GPC and CDP choline), which are often taken with Racetam derivatives. Some substances like Vinpocetine, ginkgo, Bacopa, Huperzine-A and certain modified vitamins, such as Sulbutiamine and Pyritinol (forms of vitamins B1 and B6), are often considered nootropics as well. Other natural herbs and supplements like fish oil and ginseng have been shown to positively impact memory and cognition, but aren't strictly considered nootropics. We cover these types of natural herbs and supplements towards the end of the book, in the chapter on general brain health.

Lastly, it's important to note that drugs recommended for people with narcolepsy and sleep apnea are often considered nootropics. Drugs such as Nuvigil and Provigil are examples of such prescription medications. It might be hard for you to obtain a prescription if you do not suffer from the conditions they typically treat.

Why They're Valuable

Nootropics are effective because they enhance the network of neurons in the brain that are connected by synapses. Chemicals called neurotransmitters enable these neurons to communicate and work together. A nootropic simply boosts the production of these neurotransmitters, thus greasing the wheels for more rapid and effective communication between the neurons that enable every thought and function in your brain.

Nootropics do not instantly make you a genius, but they do enable your brain to work at a higher capacity than normal. As your synapses work more efficiently, you can experience improved concentration, better memory and an increased attention span. Think of the impact of the common drug Adderall without the side effects. Nootropics can have very similar effects.

In addition to these enhanced neurotransmitters, nootropics increase the blood flow to your brain through a process called vasodiliation. With that increased bloodflow comes more oxygen and glucose, an energy source that helps your brain focus for longer periods of time. This extra energy improves one's memory and the overall function of the brain.

Studies have also shown nootropics benefit those with decreased brain function like the elderly or those who've suffered repeated concussions or traumatic brain injuries. Other studies have demonstrated nootropics ability to slow memory loss and (perhaps) even counteract the effects of Alzheimer's disease.

How They're Used

As news spreads about the benefits of Nootropics, online communities like those on Reddit and Longecity are cropping up to discuss the benefits and drawbacks of usage. Most users report positive effects from taking nootropics, but mention that the effects go away after they stop taking them (though don't experience typical addictive responses like tremors and headaches). In other words, students cramming for tests don't become geniuses once they stop taking them after exam week. Most nootropics only work for as long as they're taken.

In a recent article, *Details* magazine interviewed several nootropics users and physicians regarding the use of this new class of drugs. One section of the story focused on an engineer that had been taking a nootropic and had raved about the experience. Jonathan Reilly, 41, from Los Angeles, reports that he used to begin his workday in a fog. "I'd come into my office feeling like I had woken up at four to take someone to the airport," he said. "It took me twice as long to accomplish anything important."

Now, he maintains a crystal-clear focus beginning with his daily 8 a.m. meetings and continuing through his 12-hour workday. He also said his mood has improved substantially since starting to take Nuvigil, a drug on many Nootropic lists. "It made me feel awake for the first time," Reilly said. "I'm much more creative and much more productive. If I'm project-managing, it's like seeing the matrix. It makes it easier to put the pieces together to come up with a complete picture."

According to the article, "hard-charging professionals" are using nootropics more and more, primarily taking prescription analeptics like Nuvigil and Provigil, as well as less-potent supplements like New Mood and Alpha Brain that combine vitamins, amino acids and antioxidants.

People who take nootropics say that they differ substantially from energy drinks because they do not experience any crash or jitters. Roy Cohen, a career coach in New York City and author of *The Wall Street Professional's Survival Guide*, observed, "These drugs are used in industries where there's less room for failure and immediate results are expected. These people thrive on accomplishment—it's in their DNA.

It's incredibly seductive to have this potential for guaranteed peak performance."

Joe, a 26-year-old banking consultant in Chicago, said that he started taking Alpha Brain while getting his M.B.A. and continued its usage as he prepped for his CPA exam. "I'd retain more information than I would if I hadn't taken it," he reported. He still uses Alpha Brain before presentations and doesn't feel nervous anymore. "It gives me confidence. I feel like I'm working on my optimal levels while I'm on it."

Even with this regular use, those who take Nootropics say that they feel no ill effects if they miss a day. Many use the word "clarity" to describe how they feel when they take them. Physicians have started to prescribe Provigil and Nuvigil when their patients complain of frequent jet lag and excessive fatigue. Other users order the drugs online, though psychiatrists recommend only using nootropics with a prescription. Emily Deans, a psychiatrist in Boston, cautions patients to steer clear of Nootropics that contain Huperzine A. "This ingredient can make you more alert and sharpen thinking, but if you take too much at once, you can make yourself psychotic," she noted. "I don't know if it's ethical to recommend, but for students using it to study or surgeons trying to stay up all night long, a (prescription Nootropic) might be useful," she added. "If they were willing to not burn the candle at both ends for too long, it might help people do a better job."

This book will serve as the definitive guide for those interested in nootropics and other brain supplements. After reading this book and doing some more of your own research, you can decide if nootropics should be a part of your life. We'll examine different categories of nootropics, how to stack them for maximum benefit, and cover the existing research on these powerful substances.

Chapter Two

Nootropic Categories

It's possible to divide nootropics into any number of categories, but for the purposes of this book we'll define Primary Nootropics as more traditional nootropics – racetams, cholines and other substances physicians traditionally associate with this category. A second category includes stimulants and supplements with similar properties as nootropics. For the purposes of this book, these two categories will be called Primary Nootropics and Secondary Nootropics. We'll also cover supplements that many nootropics users tap into as they start with cognitive enhancers.

Primary Nootropics

Primary Nootropics refer to substances derived from racetams, and all have a derivation of the racetam name in them. Racetams heighten a neurotransmitters' ability to relay messages and raise the levels of glutamate and acetylcholine in the brain. Racetams also improve communication between the two hemispheres of the brain and can even protect brain cells that would otherwise be harmed by alcohol use. This class of nootropics is by far the most widely studied.

Below are the primary derivatives of racetam:

- **Piracetam:** first synthesized in 1964, it has been shown to improve general cognition in people who have suffered mental decline, particularly among aging patients. It's also been used as a study aid and cognitive enhancer. Piracetam enhances cellular membrane fluidity and helps reduce blood clotting as effectively as aspirin. It has been used to help the brain recover from alcohol abuse and improve cognition in patients that have had a stroke or have schizophrenia. Sometimes called the first official nootropic, it is best taken with water.

- **Aniracetam:** known as the relaxing racetam, aniracetam is an ampakine subset of the racetam class. It's potentially even more effective than Piracetam due to its fat-solubility. Ampakines are known to enhance attention span and alertness, and have been shown to facilitate learning and memory. Aniracetam brands include Ampamet, Memodrin and Pergamid. This racetam has a shorter half-life than piracetam and produces a mild sedative effect that can lead to drowsiness, as opposed to piracetam's the stimulating effects. Many experts in the field think of aniracetam as an updated version of piracetam.

- **Oxiracetam**: also from the racetam class, said to be more of a stimulant than piracetam and aniracetam. This type of nootropic is no longer used in clinical applications. It brings a crash along with its rush, and users often report feeling exhausted hours after the increase in clarity and speed of thought.

- **Pramiracetam**: also goes by the name Remen, Neupramir and Pramistar, pramiracetam is said to be more potent than piracetam. It's one of the latest improved derivatives of racetam.

- **Noopept**: said to help with memory recall and could be helpful in the treatment of Alzheimer's disease. Noopept has not been exhaustively tested or used for decades as piracetam and aniracetam have been.

Secondary Nootropics

Secondary Nootropics include both synthetic and natural substances, with many products combining the two. The most common secondary nootropics are listed below:

- **Armodafinil (Nuvigil):** called an analeptic and prescribed for people who are sleep deprived as a result of working odd hours, has been shown to improve daytime wakefulness. Doctors prescribe it for people with narcolepsy and sleep apnea, both of which hinder healthy sleeping patterns.

- **Modafinil (Provigil):** similar to Nuvigil in that it improves daytime wakefulness in patients that have narcolepsy, sleep apnea or odd working hours. Modafinil has fewer side effects than many former amphetamine-based stimulants, which places it in the secondary nootropics category. Modafinil is a popular drug for wakefulness, focus and clarity of thought, though some users have experienced headaches after continued use.

- **Bacopa Monnieri:** a popular, natural extract from a plant that grows in tropical climates in the water, long used in India for mental stimulation. Bacopa users report greater memory gains and enhanced cognition.

- **L-Theanine:** naturally found in green tea, L-Theanine has been shown to improve reaction time and memory, especially when used in combination with caffeine. It can cross the blood-brain barrier and promotes alpha wave production and the production of dopamine, a mood enhancer. It might also be capable of raising glutamate levels.

- **Creatine:** known more for use among bodybuilders, this organic acid might also help the brain in many ways. In a recent experiment, vegetarians and the elderly showed improved memorization ability and cognitive ability, though this mental effect is less pronounced among younger patients.

- **Rhodiola:** a plant that grows in arctic regions of the world, its root is said to increase energy, stamina, strength and mental capacity. This root has not been vetted thoroughly by the scientific community, but its extract is known to protect cells from being damaged. It has a long history as a medicinal plant, dating back to the 1st Century. Also known as "arctic root."

- **Phenibut**: a derivative of the naturally produced inhibitory neurotransmitter y-aminobutyric acid (GABA), Phenibut is sometimes sold under the name Noofen and was developed in Russia. It is sold there as a psychotropic drug but has not been approved as a pharmaceutical in the U.S. or Europe. Studies on its effect as a Nootropic have been mixed.

- **Linopirdine**: disinhibits acetylcholine release in the brain and is being studied for use with people who have memory loss.

- **Physostigmine**: has short-term effects and has been used to treat patients with Alzheimer's disease as well as patients with traumatic brain injuries.

- **Sabeluzole**: has been shown to improve memory.

- **Pyritinol**: a semi-synthetic form of vitamin B6, it helps with glucose uptake in the brain when it is under extended strain, thus giving the brain continuous energy to perform. This improves concentration and cognitive ability.

- **Acetylcarnitine**: also known as ALCAR, it is an acetylated form of L-carnitine, which is produced by the body and used to transport fatty acids to be broken down. Some research has suggested that it could be effective in the treatment of Parkinson's disease, although it is not routinely prescribed for benefit to the brain.

Stacked Supplements

Stacked supplements are combinations of different supplements and nootropics offered by different companies on the market. Several of the most popular are below:

- **New Mood**: a combination of vitamin B6, serotonin, amino acids and antioxidants, all purported to stimulate brain receptors.

- **Alpha Brain**: contains Vinpocetine, vitamin B6, Theanine and said to raise acetylcholine levels, which are crucial to brain functioning. One of the most popular brain foods on the market. Some users have reported particularly lucid dreaming after taking Alpha Brain.

- **truBRAIN**: another very popular brain food, builds primarily on piracetam, an acknowledged nootropic, as well as DCP-Choline. Also contains Pramiracetam, another derivative from the racetam family, as well as Theanine.

- **Excelerol**: another substance that combines many vitamins and nutrients, primarily vitamin B12, along with tea extracts, Vinpocetine, and agents that will increase choline levels in the brain. Also contains Huperzine and Gingko Biloba, long reputed to increase cerebral circulation by increasing use of glucose in the brain, although some studies have shown it to have no effect on healthy males.

Below is a chart summarizing the classifications of Nootropics and their primary benefits:

PRIMARY NOOTROPICS	COMPOSITION/EFFECTS
Piracetam	Shown to improve general cognition in people who have suffered cognitive decline, e.g., aging patients. Also has been taken as a study aid and cognitive enhancer. Has also been found to reduce the number of breath-holding spells that children sometimes suffer from. Has been used to help the brain recover from alcoholism, improve cognition in patients that have had a stroke or have schizophrenia. Best taken with water.
Aniracetam	Said to be even more effective than Piracetam due to it being lipid-soluble, considered an updated version of Piracetam and known as "the relaxing Racetam." Sold under the names of Ampamet, Memodrin and Pergamid. Has a shorter half-life than Piracetam and produces a mild sedation that can lead to sleepiness, as opposed to the stimulant effect that Piracetam has. Seems to be particularly synergistic with Piracetam. Fat-soluble and thus best taken with milk.
Oxiracetam	Said to be more of a stimulant than Piracetam and Aniracetam, no longer used in clinical applications. Brings a "crash" along with its rush, with users often reporting a tiredness a couple of hours after an increase in clarity and speed of thought. Can also make the user feel detached from what s/he is doing.
Pramiracetam	Also goes by the names of Remen, Neupramir and Pramistar, said to be more potent than Piracetam.
	Said to help with memory recall and could be helpful in

	the treatment of Alzheimer's disease. Has not been exhaustively tested or used for decades as Piracetam and Aniracetam have been, so should be used with caution.
SECONDARY NOOTROPICS	
Armodafinil (Nuvigil)	Termed an analeptic and prescribed for people who are sleep deprived as a result of working odd hours, has been shown to improve daytime wakefulness. Also prescribed for people with narcolepsy and sleep apnea, both of which hinder healthy sleeping patterns.
Modafinil (Provigil)	Similar to Nuvigil in that it improves daytime wakefulness in patients that have narcolepsy, sleep apnea or odd working hours. Has fewer side effects than many former amphetamine-based stimulants. Said to regulate the histamine levels of the brain to charge it as needed.
Linopirdine	Disinhibits acetylcholine release in the brain, being studied for use with people who have loss of memory.
Physostigmine	Has short-term effects and has been used to treat patients with Alzheimer's disease as well as patients with traumatic brain injuries.
Salubezole	Has been proven to improve memory, found in many of the Nootropics in this chart.

Pyritinol	Semi-synthetic form of vitamin B6, helps with glucose uptake in the brain when it is under extended strain, thus giving the brain continuous energy to perform.
Bacopa Monnieri	Extract from a plant that grows in tropical climates in the water, long used in India for mental stimulation; users of this report greater memory gains and enhanced cognition.
L-Theanine	Found in green tea and isolated for inclusion in many types of foods and beverages, especially in Japan. When used in combination with caffeine, undoubtedly improves reaction time and memory. Able to cross the blood-brain barrier and promotes alpha wave production and the production of dopamine, a mood enhancer. Might also be capable of raising glutamate levels.
Creatine	Known for years in the bodybuilding community as a muscle builder, this organic acid produced in the body to give energy to muscles might also have a beneficent effect on the brain. Tests on vegetarians and the elderly showed strong increase in cognitive ability; tests on young people showed no gains.
	Also sold under the brand name Noofen, Phenibut is a supplement developed in Russia, not approved as a

	pharmaceutical in the U.S. or Europe yet. A derivative of the inhibitory neurotransmitter y-aminobutyric acid, or GABA. Studies of its effectiveness as a Nootropic are mixed.
Acetylcarnitine	Also known as ALCAR, an acetylated form of L-carnitine, which is produced by the body and used to transport fatty acids to be broken down. Some research has suggested that it could be effective in the treatment of Parkinson's disease, although it is not routinely prescribed for benefit to the brain.
Rhodiola	Also known as "arctic root," referring o where it's grown, this plant's root is said to increase energy, stamina, strength and mental capacity, with potential for improved learning and memory. These claims are based primarily on evidence that its extract protects cells in the body. It has a long history as a medicinal plant, dating back to the 1st Century.
Stacked Supplements	
New Mood	A combination of vitamin B6, serotonin, amino acids and antioxidants, all purported to stimulate brain receptors.
	Contains Vinpocetine, vitamin B6, Theanine, reputed to raise acetylcholine levels, which are crucial to brain

	functioning. One of the most popular brain foods on the market. Some users have reported particularly lucid dreaming after taking Alpha Brain.
truBRAIN	Another very popular brain food, builds primarily on Piracetam, as well as DCP-Choline, which is used in stacking with Piracetam in many cases. Represents a stacking of Nootropics in one packet. Also contains Pramiracetam, another derivative from the Racetam family, as well as Theanine.
Excelerol	Another substance that combines many vitamins and nutrients, primarily vitamin B12, along with tea extracts, Vinpocetine, and agents that will increase choline levels in the brain. Also contains Huperzine and Gingko Biloba, long reputed to increase cerebral circulation by increasing use of glucose in the brain.
MindRx	Similar formula to Excelerol, with Choline, Vinpocetine and Gingko Biloba.
Neuro1	Also builds off B12, Piracetam, Gingko Biloba, Vinpocetine, Huperzine A and Theanine, as well as caffeine. The inclusion of Piracetam differentiates this substance from others with similar blends.
	Said to be a "natural" alternative to Adderall. Builds off Vitamin B3 and contains Choline, Vinpocetine and

	Huperzine. Acknowledged as a stimulant, eliminating it from the Primary Nootropic category. Also said to reduce body fat!
Illuminal	Said to be a mood-lifter and energy-giver, building off B6 and B12 vitamins, acetyl-L Carnitine and Sulbutiamine, a semi-synthetic form of vitamin B1 that helps with the modulation of dopamine in the brain, which improves mood and gives a sensation of well-being.

Visit http://thenootropicsbook.com/stacks for resources about where you can buy these different supplements, as well as receive a guide for how to create a personalized nootropics stack.

Chapter Three

Stacking Nootropics

When nootropic users refer to "stacking," they mean taking various nootropic substances to amplify their effects. One definition of stacking from an experienced nootropics user goes like this: "A stack simply involves any pairing of substances that enhance and complement each other when taken simultaneously."

With that definition in mind, it should be noted that many pills and powders already stack a variety of substances reputed to increase brain function. That would make it even more prudent for users of Nootropics to be wary of stacking these substances together. Think of taking two products off of the list of secondary nootropics in chapter two and you can imagine the exponential effect of taking two pre-stacked products. Would that give you more focus and energy? Probably not.

A third definition of stacking would apply when a person buys a bulk raw powder of a given Nootropic and mixes his own capsules to create a formula that will give him the greatest desired effect. People deeply into the study of Nootropics might feel qualified to mix their own batches of Nootropics, but it's probably not a good idea for the beginner.

The Most Common Form of Nootropic Stacking

The most popular stacks involve mixing Choline with one of the primary nootropics listed in the previous chapter. This is because taking certain nootropics can up your brain's requirement for choline, as the brain ramps production and output. It's as if nootropics run your brain at a higher horsepower, requiring more gasoline that choline supplements provide. A water-soluble nutrient, choline helps to keep cell membranes healthy and serves as the precursor for the neurotransmitter acetylcholine, which governs memory and muscle control. Some research indicates that that many people do not consume enough choline, with as few as 10% of people receiving enough of this important nutrient.

Even without use in concert with Nootropics, Choline can

increase a person's cognitive ability. A 2011 study in the *American Journal of Clinical Nutrition* found that higher Choline intake resulted in better verbal and visual memory, as well as improved verbal learning over a period of four years. The increased Choline intake also limited brain atrophy. This substance has also been shown in lab tests to improve memory, and it has long been known that it plays an important role in the production of new brain cells.

Common Choline supplements include Choline Bitartrate and Choline Citrate, said to be very helpful for people with racetam-induced headaches. Some nootropics users eat foods high in Choline, such as eggs. Others up their defense against headaches by increasing their intake of Omega-3 fish oil.

Studies on rats have shown that Choline combined with Piracetam results in vastly improved brain function. The rats, which had shown some brain deterioration, did slightly better when given Piracetam, but when given Piracetam and Choline together, they exhibited retention scores several times better.

Citicoline – also known as CDP-Choline – is another source of choline. It has been shown to slow the brain deterioration that comes with Alzheimer's disease. It also increases one's dopamine level, which can result in a more positive mood.

L-Alpha Glycerylphosphorylcholine, also known as Alpha GPC, is one of the more potent forms of Choline. It can be found in dairy products but occurs most often in purified soy Lecithin. Choline Bitartrate, also known as Choline Salt, is easily available and often used in used in nootropic stacks.

Other foods with high levels of Choline include liver, turkey heart, egg yolk, caribou meat, quinoa, bacon and milk products. Vegetables, unfortunately, do not have much Choline, and vegetarians can suffer from a lack of Choline intake.

For suggested nootropic stacks for both beginners and advanced users, check out our resources page at http://thenootropicsbook.com/stacks.

Chapter Four

Medical Evidence for Nootropics

As with any new classification of drugs, it takes time for appropriate research to be done and for the medical community to issue a verdict on the given substance regarding its safety and efficacy. The current fascination with "brain food" is not new; researchers have been testing cognitive enhancers for decades, but almost all of that testing has been with subjects that have had serious brain issues. The aim of most Nootropics research to this point has been to see if they can reverse the effects of aging and/or help people who have suffered brain injuries to recover most or all of their normal functioning. In other words, scant clinical research has been done on the effect of Nootropics on healthy individuals because that body of research has not been a priority in the medical community.

Logically, one would assume that if Nootropics can reverse some aspects of memory loss or enable elderly patients to concentrate for longer periods of time, they would have a similarly beneficial effect on healthy individuals. This chapter will take a look at the research and let the reader decide if obtaining these drugs and substances would be a wise move or folly.

Normal people with healthy brain function have become much more interested in nootropics and other cognitive enhancers because they sense a need to gain some sort of mental edge at their school and/or workplace. Unfortunately, there has not been much research conducted on the impact of these cognitive enhancers on healthy brains. Fortunately, no researchers have found that taking Nootropics or other cognitive enhancers has had a negative impact on a healthy person.

As authorities at the University of Washington stated: "Although there are many companies that make 'smart' drinks, smart power bars and diet supplements containing 'smart' chemicals, there is little evidence to suggest that these products really work ... There are very few well-designed studies using normal healthy people... The strongest evidence for these substances is for the improvement of cognitive function in people with brain injury or disease (for example, Alzheimer's disease and traumatic brain injury)."

This area of research rests on the solid foundation that nootropics increase the level of Choline in the brain, which repairs and enhances the neurotransmitter acetylcholine. Researchers concentrating on the reversal of the symptoms of Alzheimer's disease are discussing two approaches to helping those who suffer from it, either increasing levels of acetylcholine or slowing the death of neurons that contain acetylcholine. Nootropics such as Piracetam could probably help in this quest; they seem to enhance the production of acetylcholine, and users often stack them with Choline supplements that definitely boost acetylcholine amounts in the brain.

Vinpocetine, found in many Nootropic stacks, also reduces brain cell loss and increase both blood flow and the efficiency of the use of glucose to power the brain. Vinpocetine has passed many lab tests with sterling results.

A Summary of Several Studies of Nootropics

Effects of Piracetam and Piracetam-like Drugs on Central Nervous System (CNS) Disorders

This review of all of the literature in this area looked at studies done in the past decade or so and zeroed in on these central nervous system disorders: a) cognition/memory; b) epilepsy and seizure; c) neurodegenerative diseases; d) stroke/ischaemia; e) stress and anxiety.

Several Nootropics performed quite well in these studies. Pramiracetam improved cognitive deficits associated with traumatic brain injuries. Piracetam has been shown to have a welcome protective effect when used during coronary bypass surgery and was effective in treating CNS disorders that involved cerebrovascular and traumatic origins.

Piracetam did not seem to have long-term benefits, however, for those who had what were termed "mild" cognitive impairments. Its most prominent effect was on lowering depression and anxiety, more so than for improving memory. Piracetam appeared to have stronger impacts on cognitive disabilities when used in conjunction with other drugs, perhaps a good argument for nootropic stacking.

Neural Ramifications of Nootropic drugs in the Healthy Developing Brain

This recent study has been one of the most significant of its kind, both in scope and detail. It has many important findings that potential users of Nootropics should take into consideration. Performed by two professors in departments of psychology and neurobiology and anatomy, the study either repeated earlier findings or broke new ground with these conclusions:

- Any substance that can be classified as a stimulant will help the memory/learning circuits of the brain. Any substance that boosts production of dopamine, glutamate or norepinephrine will "improve brain function in healthy individuals beyond their baseline functioning."

- With the gain in memory/learning abilities provided by stimulants comes a few dangers, chiefly a large alteration in the function of glutamate in the brain, which can impair behavioral flexibility. In laymen's terms, that means that it can be very easy to become addicted to these stimulants. This risk is especially high among adolescents and young adults.

- Modafinil, also known as Provigil, bears a close resemblance to methylphenidate (MPH), a stimulant that did not fare well in testing because it negatively affects other forms of higher reasoning. Developed in France in the 1970s, Modafinil elevates histamine levels in the brain, although its mechanism of action has not been clearly established. Modafinil has been approved by the U.S. Food and Drug Administration (FDA) for treatment of narcolepsy, shift-work disorder and obstructive sleep apnea. It also has been proven to help with jet lag and positive emotions, helping shift workers that often struggle with depression related to chronic fatigue. Modafinil has become a popular alternative to amphetamines to keep soldiers awake and alert for long periods of time in potentially high-stress situations.

- As Modafinil gains a reputation as a Nootropic that is safer than other stimulants, it could begin to quickly gain ground on a variety of substances that improve wakefulness and concentration. However, Modafinil has been shown to cause dizziness, anxiety, agitation and insomnia in younger children. The exact cut-off point for when a person's body can handle Modafinil easily without these side effects has not been established, although the FDA has approved it for use in children aged 16 and over. No one knows what will happen if Modafinil becomes the latest wonder drug for cramming students in high schools across the country.

- Modafinil's inclusion on the list of Nootropics and/or cognitive enhancers contains some merit. Modafinil "induces improvements in pattern recognition memory, digit span recall and mental digit manipulation (performing addition/subtraction/multiplication in one's mind)." Gains in spatial memory, attention and other executive functioning were more ambiguous, with gains coming largely in persons of low

IQ.

- Dangers associated with Modafinil resemble the dangers listed about other stimulants. It could very well affect logical thinking and decision making in users under the age of 30, when the front of the brain matures to its maximum. Teens are particularly at risk, and could face very difficult alterations in their sleep cycles and motivational levels. As the portion of the study focusing on Modafinil concluded, "Future studies will need to address these shortcomings in order to determine the safety and efficacy of Modafinil as a true cognitive enhancer."

- Ampakines, such as Aniracetam, continue to rapidly evolve from drugs for the treatment of Alzheimer's disease to usage as a cognitive enhancer, with the same sorts of cautions for young users as other Nootropics. Scientists are studying Ampakines for use with patients having Parkinson's disease, ADHD, Rhett's syndrome, schizophrenia, depression and autism. Obviously, with that list of foes, of they prove to be effective, they will enjoy a wide market of use. Ampakines have been proven to improve memory and cognition in both humans and rats.

- Ampakines become potentially quite attractive to those who want to use a cognitive enhancer because they do not stimulate the central nervous system, one reason why Aniracetam made it onto the list of Primary Nootropics in the previous chapter. Some evidence has surfaced of Ampakines causing headaches and nausea.

- Again, young users of Ampakines could face several undesirable consequences, among them "poor emotional regulation and impaired behavioral inhibition." In scientific terms, Ampakines strengthen all of the brain's synapses, thus the weaker synapses are not pruned, and overload can result, where a person cannot process all of the stimulation coming to the brain. As the researchers stated, "The signal-to-noise ratio is greatly lowered," meaning that people who take high doses of Ampakines could develop "autism-like syndromes." "Careful determination of a dose-response curve, toxic effects and species differences in metabolism/reaction to Ampakines will need to be completed in the future in order to determine their true utility as cognitive enhancers," researchers concluded.

Scientific Findings and User Testimonials

When wading through the extravagant claims of any number of products on the Internet or even in a health food store, it can be difficult to determine truth from fiction. One should also be wary of fads that come into vogue and then fade away as the dangers of a given product, or simply their unreliability, come to light.

Nootropic drugs have been tested and discussed for more than 40 years, yet most recent researchers agree that much more testing needs to be done to determine exactly how powerful these drugs are. That said, a few seemingly objective reviews of Nootropic drugs can be found online. One was from an article written for *The Atlantic* magazine, titled "Experimenting with Nootropics to Improve Mental Capacity, Clarity." In this article, writer Ari Levaux gave a detailed account of his journey with the Alpha Brain supplement, which contains Vinpocetine and Theanine, two heavyweight substances that have a proven impact on the brain. Theanine is found in tea and has long been hailed for its mildly stimulating properties, while Vinpocetine is a synthetic substance that increases blood flow to the brain and protects brain cells.

Levaux said that he did not feel any effect from the mix until he was falling asleep, at which time he "monitored the entire process and remained lucid, with a measure of free will, as I dreamed, and woke up surprisingly refreshed." He went on to share that "Alpha Brain's most noticeable impact ... was making it easier to wake up early. Since I'm typically not a morning person, this was striking, and helpful. I also felt slightly more organized, and a curious sense of emotional stability."

Levaux contacted Alpha Brain's manufacturers and discovered that his enhanced dreaming was due to the product's ability to boost acetylcholine, due to its two primary ingredients: GPC Choline and Huperzine A. "Huperzine A disarms the enzyme that naturally breaks down acetylcholine. So while the GPC Choline is being converted to acetylcholine, the Huperzine A is keeping it from disappearing. It's like plugging the drain and turning on the faucet," the company's CEO told him.

Levaux also called a clinical psychiatrist who teaches at Harvard Medical School to discuss his hunting trip while on Alpha Brain. She responded by saying that there was "probably nothing dangerous" about the occasional use of nootropics for specific time frames with a need for elevated concentration, such as finals week or before a large project was due. However, she added, it could be possible to build up a tolerance to such drugs over time and recommended sticking to pharmaceutical-grade products that could be accurately dosed and less likely to be contaminated. She also said that if one's acetylcholine level is too high, if the faucet is turned up too strongly, then the nervous system can be impacted, with heart rate, blood pressure and even temperature affected.

Levaux's final advice to those looking for the next super drug? "The number of neuroactive products being studied and brought to market today is unprecedented, and it's tempting to think some of these might make you a more effective person. Explore carefully. With

Nootropics, due diligence is in order."

The top search engine result for "Nootropics Testimonials" lands one on the page of Jonathan Roseland, who publishes a site called "Limitless Mind." While not specifying the ingredients in the Nootropics cocktail that he imbibed, he did credit it with helping him to find an accounting error that he would have usually missed. "Can I credit all my attention to detail, discipline and general coolness under fire to the smart drugs flowing in my veins?" Roseland asked. "That's hard to say for sure. I've had enough moments while on Nootropics that my focus, attention and creativity either saved the day or delivered the rock star results that people pay me the big bucks for." He then went on to rank different Nootropics based on testimonials, money-back guarantees and other factors. His report of reviews on Amazon, if you value such numbers, ranked the Nootropics mentioned in this book in this order:

1. Alpha Brain

2. Neuro1

3. Excelerol

4. Iluminal

5. Addrena

6. Mind Power Rx

Another regular user of Nootropics tried an extensive range of the drugs and gave detailed accounts of his experiences. He ranked the Nootropics that he tried in this order of effectiveness:

1. Modafinil

2. Melatonin

3. Caffeine and Theanine

4. Piracetam and Choline

5. Vitamin D

6. Sulbutiamine

7. Fish Oil

This particular reviewer made this interesting comment about Nootropics: "I view Nootropics as akin to a biological lottery; one good discovery pays for all." His comments seemed to echo many other reviewers, in that the perceived effects of a stimulant are always greater than the purest nootropics out of the racetam family. Because nootropics from the racetam family do not have an instant result, it can be difficult to measure their impact right away.

Another popular review can be found on the Longecity website, where one person condensed 10 months of personal "research" into a brief outline of the effects of certain nootropics on his brain, body and life.

This researcher stacked Nootropics with caffeine and said that he was "able to study for the bar exam all day with zero mental fatigue." He also reported that he could "read vast quantities of information only one time and spit it back with pinpoint precision," which fits with several of the reputed benefits of nootropics: increased memory and reduction of mental fatigue. Of his regimen, he mentioned that "It is the closest thing to a photographic memory I have ever experienced."

The wonder cocktail that this user recommended consisted of piracetam, CDP Choline and either Sulbutiamine or Pyritinol. The latter two substances reportedly reduce mental fatigue and increase overall alertness, giving the same effect in essence, meaning that either was acceptable as the third element in this stack. Other supplements he recommended were Aniracetam, fish oil and Bacopa, all of which we covered earlier in the book. Aniracetam, a more potent version of Piracetam, must be taken in smaller quantities than its parent, with this user recommending 4000 mg of Piracetam and 750 mg of Aniracetam daily. He recommended diversifying nootropics intake to draw on different mechanisms for increased cognitive functioning. He also reminded users that the effects were cumulative, not short term, and that users would see greater gains on day 91 than day 1.

The nootropic sub-group on Reddit.com has numerous testimonials every day, some positive, some negative and others neutral. One noteworthy recent testimonial touched on a common theme when discussing Piracetam, that its effect is both subtle and cumulative. One user stacked Piracetam with two doses of Adafrinil and saw quick and obvious results. "Never felt so motivated and productive and efficient in my life." As his body adjusted to Adafrinil, he moved to Addrena. He reported mixed results with this combo, saying that some days he was wired but mentally foggy, while on others he experienced heightened clarity.

Some of the reviewers of Nootropics have actually compiled the experiences of others on their sites, as well as dug up hard-to-find research on testing involving Nootropics on healthy individuals, which can be helpful even though the sample sizes are small.

A quick look at some of these studies, many of them done in Europe, yields these findings:

- Healthy individuals in a study done in Scandinavia improved their mental performance with the use of Piracetam. It also helped improve learning in children with learning disorders, such as Dyslexia, and boosted brainpower in undernourished rats. The best results with this substance were achieved when taken over seven consecutive days, reinforcing the idea that the racetam family of drugs does not produce an instantaneous feeling of euphoria or alertness.

- Piracetam and Aniracetam reduced drug-induced cognitive impairments, a consistent finding for nootropics.

- Oxiracetam also reduced the impairments of drug-induced

states and improved memory, learning and attention.

- Pramiracetam joined the other members of the racetam family in reducing impairments caused by drugs.

- Choline improved the effectiveness in Piracetam, proving the wisdom of stacking with Choline.

When all is said and done, the decision to use nootropics rests with the individual and what s/he wants to accomplish through usage of these drugs. The strictest category of nootropics have absolutely done wonders for the damaged brains of many, and they may find broader application with people who have suffered concussions and children with learning disabilities. Users of the racetam family of drugs do not always report monumental changes in their mental acuity, but they probably have not given the drugs long enough to have their effect.

Many of what this book has termed "Secondary Nootropics" do have a multitude of fans, many of who have felt the effects of a stimulant and thus have experienced a greater and longer-lasting ability to concentrate during a given time period. If you seek that type of boost, a Secondary Nootropic might be your best bet.

In short, Nootropics have not been found to damage anyone's brain, and the narrowest category of these smart drugs earn their places on the short lists precisely because they do not have many side effects and they are not addictive. In other words, if you try a nootropic or stack with nootropics, you might not sense any remarkable change in your mental abilities, but you could sense an improved clarity.

Nootropics present a low-risk but sometimes expensive opportunity to improve your brain's functioning over the short or long term. An abundance of first-person accounts on the Web cover just about every combination you can imagine of nootropics. Your brain is probably not an organ that you want to experiment too extensively on, but if you desire an uptick in your mental game, nootropics present little harm and possible help.

Researchers have definitively proven that nootropics improve brain functioning, and abundant user testimonials affirm their positive effect on clarity, memory, processing and other cognitive functions. Many of those users appreciate that nootropics have negligible side effects and are non-addictive, although once a user stops taking them, they often revert to their previous state. Many of the nootropics mentioned in this e-book have had all of the positive effects of long-used stimulants, without the crash afterwards. The vast majority of user testimonials show a definitive, positive effect, and it can be very difficult to find a testimonial that reports unwanted side effects of any type. As research on these exciting new drugs continues, it will be fascinating to see if they can grow and heal our brains in ways that we do not yet imagine. That will be spectacularly good news not just for Alzheimer's patients, but also for the millions of modern people who want to tap their brain's capacity to the fullest.

Chapter 5

Keys to Better Brain Health

The requirements of modern life demand that our brains work at a very high level with no allowance for days passed in a mental fog. We cannot thrive in a wired world if our brain is continually tired and lagging. As a result, the medical community has pumped up its study of the brain, and the advances in this area could be the most stunning of the 21st Century.

Along with increased research on nootropics has also come increased analysis of how the brain works in varying conditions. As you do your own research on mental fitness, three elements appear again and again in the literature for maximum brain function: exercise, brain-friendly foods and time reserved for meditation or reflection.

Exercise and the Brain

Studies have shown that our body actually works together with our brain and is meant to engage in movement on a daily basis. The most recent studies on brain health have not focused drugs or supplements to help the brain, but on the supporting cast of the brain—the muscles and joints that move the body and release all sorts of great chemicals within the brain. Our body needs balance, not just mental exercise, but physical recreation as well. It is one unit and works best in a fascinating combination of movement and mental effort.

Furthermore, regular, vigorous exercise enables a person to sleep better, an absolutely essential activity for anyone that wants to increase brain capacity. A lack of sleep will do more to inhibit your brain's functioning that almost any other type of activity that you can think of, outside of taking various toxic drugs and substances. People who exercise sleep more deeply and more easily for longer periods of time, ensuring optimal alertness during the hours they are awake.

Here are several recent findings on this intriguing relationship between the brain and exercise:

- Women over 65 who walked 30 minutes a day slowed their cognitive decline.

- A more active group of seniors over 70 was far less likely to develop cognitive problems than one that was not active. Even standing up and walking around a room was found to be beneficial!

- People who exercise have larger brains. MRIs have borne this out, a critical measure as brains decrease in size with age.

- Exercise uses more brain cells, which turns on genes that make brain-derived neurotropic factor (BDNF), which rewires memory circuits. Researchers urged five days of exercise per week to see these types of benefits.

Brain-Friendly Foods

Antioxidants not only help to fight off cancer and other toxic enemies, they reduce signs of aging in the brain and can even increases its size. Foods loaded with omega-3 fatty acids are particularly helpful in the quest to have a vigorous brain. These include:

- Bluberries, cranberries and raspberries

- Fish

- Nuts and seeds

- Artichokes

- Prunes

- Sage

- Rosemary

- Turmeric

- Ginger

Meditation/Reflection

Scientists at UCLA have found that meditation increases the folding in the cerebral cortex, effectively changing the brain's architecture, which improves its ability to process information. This folding, also called cortical gyrification, enables us to retrieve memories, make decisions and focus on one task at a time.

In addition, meditation has long been known to reduce stress, which can block the neural circuits of the brain and keep it from achieving its maximum productivity. Meditation calms many areas of the brain and enables it to process and block stress more vigorously, enabling the circuits to thrive unimpeded.

A Final Word

Just because you take nootropics does not mean that you should not exercise, sleep, eat right and set aside quiet time for reflection. Similarly, doing all of the right things to help your brain does not preclude you from taking nootropics to see if you can achieve an even higher level of mental acuity. The recommended approach would combine finding the right nootropic combination for you, but also exercising, eating well and breathing "off the grid" from time to time to do all that you can to use your most precious organ.

The most carefully defined nootropics are non-addictive and do not usually bring side effects. They can be a great addition to your daily routine if you sense the need for greater focus, memory, processing or simple alertness. Other stimulants can be addictive and should be carefully consumed in nootropic stacking. Do your research, talk to friends, examine medical studies and experiment carefully with the proper mix of nootropics that help you to achieve the state of mental sharpness that you seek.

Chapter 6

The Future of Nootropics

As medical research expands into the use of nootropics' effects on healthy brains and additional studies are done on how to slow dreaded diseases such as Alzheimer's and Parkinson's, the future shines very brightly for rapid advances in this area of pharmacology. In addition, research done on depression has also proven promising for possible development of future synthetic nootropics that can help everyone think and process information better, not just be relieved of depression.

Two particular standouts that have recently splashed onto the scene are GLYX-13 and NSI-189. Both sound like great titles for science fiction movies or crime serials on television, but they represent the new wave of nootropics that could become huge hits in the very near future.

GLYX-13

This compound has been tested for use on patients with major depressive disorder (MDD). Initial results indicate very effective relief of depression with a high tolerance by users, with the reviews so positive that some are hailing this substance as a "major breakthrough for patients suffering from depression."

That's good news, but the even better news came from an NIH study on the N-methyl-D-aspartate receptor modulator's (NMDAR) reaction to GLYX-13 on young adult and aging rats, which revealed that it enhanced learning and memory in those test animals. The NMDAR is a key part of the brain, showing decline as aging sets in and significantly altered when the brains of those with Alzheimer's disease are examined. GLYX-13 has been shown to act as "a NMDAR receptor partial agonist … with therapeutic potential as a cognitive enhancer." GLYX-13 crosses the blood brain barrier and has boosted learning and memory in both young and aging rats. These positive outcomes have generated a strong buzz in the scientific community; stay tuned for the development of this substance.

Similarly, NSI-189 has been applied to people suffering from MDD but has also shown to aid the brain with memory and learning. In short, the research on treating depression has shifted from a focus on brain chemicals to growing and protecting brain cells as a block to depression, a change from brain chemistry mixing to brain physiology alteration. That has resulted in possible additions to the Nootropics family as these substances are used outside of the MDD sufferers' community.

The hippocampus in the brain produces neural stem cells. Drugs that can boost the hippocampus' ability to produce these cells, which produce neurons, will aid not only those who suffer from depression, but possibly those whose brains are decaying. In a question parallel to others posed in this e-book, experts on Nootropics now wonder if a boost in neural stem cells will also help those who want greater brain efficiency, not simply those who are aging or have suffered brain trauma.

Initial tests of NSI-13 showed "clinically meaningful" improvement of depression and higher scores on cognitive measures.

Researchers were especially pleased by the sustained gains made by participants in the tests thanks to NSI-13.

The next goal for the drug's developers is to stimulate growth of the hippocampus to the point where patients could eventually stop taking the drug, talking even of a "cure" for depression by reviving the hippocampus to lifelong expansion. These observations are based at this point on experiments on rats and chimpanzees, but increased testing on humans will continue as well. As for the impact on healthy brains if a hippocampus is grown to an extra-large size? The lead researcher says, "It's an exciting possibility and we'll definitely be looking out for it."

Again, stay tuned for research results on NSI-13, another drug that might become one of the most effective brain boosters of all.

Chapter 7

Conclusion

I hope you've gotten a sense of how powerful these brain

supplements and nootropics can be when it comes to improving mental

performance. To stay up to date with the latest research, find

trustworthy suppliers and to receive a free guide to making your own

nootropics stack, check out our resources at

http://thenootropicsbook.com.

SOURCES

http://nootriment.com/what-are-nootropics/#sthash.D2JmMx1W.dpuf

http://thenootropicsguide.com/what-are-nootropics/

http://www.ncbi.nlm.nih.gov/pubmed/9260731

http://www.ncbi.nlm.nih.gov/pubmed/20166767

http://www.ncbi.nlm.nih.gov/pubmed/2690149

http://www.ncbi.nlm.nih.gov/pmc/articles/PMC3035742/

http://examine.com/supplements/Piracetam/

http://www.details.com/health-fitness/diet/201305/nootropics-smart-drugs-pills

https://faculty.washington.edu/chudler/smartd.html

JEP-35326-effectiveness-of--cholinergic-nootropics-to-improve-cognitiv_121112.pdf

http://www.purenootropics.net/beginners-guide-choline/

http://www.brainsupplementstutor.com/beginners-guide-to-nootropics/

http://www.thehackedmind.com/the-ultimate-guide-to-nootropics/

http://www.theatlantic.com/health/archive/2012/01/experimenting-with-nootropics-to-increase-mental-capacity-clarity/252162/

http://www.limitlessmindset.com/mind-power-products/45-which-brain-supplements-nootropics-are-the-most-credible-limitless-pill-like-smart-drugs.html

http://journal.frontiersin.org/Journal/10.3389/fnsys.2014.00038/full

http://www.gwern.net/Nootropics

http://peaknootropics.com/list-nootropic-studies-healthy-people/

http://www.longecity.org/forum/topic/36691-ten-months-of-research-condensed-a-total-newbies-guide-to-nootropics/

http://www.reddit.com/r/Nootropics/comments/27xniv/my_brain_enhancing_story_incomplete/

http://www.huffingtonpost.com/maria-rodale/the-3-keys-to-a-healthy-b_b_3383382.html

http://www.health.harvard.edu/press_releases/regular-exercise-releases-brain-chemicals-key-for-memory-concentration-and-mental-sharpness

http://sebastianmarshall.com/my-experiences-with-modafinil

CPSIA information can be obtained at www.ICGtesting.com
Printed in the USA
LVOW04s1504211214

419839LV00033B/1492/P

9 781502 583871